AN END TO INFERTILITY :
The Ultimate Guide on Causes, Symptoms, and Treatment of infertility

Ashly Larkins

Table of content

Chapter 1

What is infertility?

Infertility is the inability of a man or female to conceive as a result of an issue with either partner's reproductive system.

Types of infertility

Primary infertility

Secondary infertility

When a person is completely unable to conceive, it is primary infertility. Someone who has previously conceived but is no longer able to do so with secondary infertility.

This page describes infertility's causes, kinds, and treatments in addition to additional information concerning infertility in both sexes that a reader could find interesting.

Most people at some point in their lives will have a strong desire to become parents. Knowing what constitutes normal fertility is essential for assisting an individual or couple in determining when assistance is needed. The majority of couples (around 85%) will become pregnant after trying for a year, with the earlier months having the highest chance of conception. Only 7% more couples will get pregnant in the second year. Infertility has come to be regarded as the inability to conceive within a year. Therefore, 15% of couples trying to conceive share this diagnosis. In general, if conception has not occurred within a year, we advise consulting a reproductive endocrinologist.

Situations for early medical help:

1)Infrequent menstrual cycles: A woman nearly always ovulates regularly when she experiences regular menstrual cycles, which are defined as cycles that occur every 21 to 35 days. The egg ovulates around two weeks before the beginning of the following menstruation. A woman may not be ovulating an egg predictably or even at all if her periods are spaced apart by more than 35 days. Egg ovulation is necessary for pregnancy. Therefore, if a couple trying to conceive has irregular or infrequent menstrual periods, we advise getting them evaluated.

2)Female age of 35 years or older: For unknown causes, egg production declines quickly as women get older. Egg quality, or the probability that an egg will be gene the lady has had a pelvic infection in the past. We will do an HSG as part of the fertility assessment to determine whether the fallopian tubes are opentically normal, and also declines with age. Therefore, if a couple has been trying to conceive for six months or more and the woman is 35 years of age or older, we advise having her fertility evaluated.

3)A background of sexually transmitted illnesses or pelvic infections: The fallopian tubes may become inflamed and permanently scarred as a result of STDs like gonorrhea or chlamydia. For natural conception to occur, there must be open tubes because sperm needs to travel through them to reach and fertilize the ovulated egg. We advise pregnancies being attempted by a couple to undergo prompt examination if the lady has had a pelvic infection in the past. We will do an HSG as part of the fertility assessment to determine whether the fallopian tubes are open.

4)Endometrial polyps or uterine fibroids: Endometrial polyps and fibroids that indent the endometrial cavity are examples of uterine abnormalities that might interfere with the interaction between the endometrium and the embryo, lowering the likelihood of implantation and pregnancy. Additionally, these anomalies may result in irregular menstrual flow. Women having a history of these abnormalities or intermenstrual bleeding should undergo evaluation after six months of trying to get pregnant. The primary method for treating or eliminating these uterine anomalies is hysteroscopy, a surgical procedure that involves inserting a small scope with a camera within the uterus cavity. The surgeon might use instruments inserted through the hysteroscope to remove or treat any anatomical anomalies.

Tests for infertility

1)Physical examination and history - Your fertility doctor will first and foremost conduct a very detailed medical and fertility history. Many of the following inquiries may be posed to you by your doctor: How long have you been attempting to conceive? How often do you engage in sexual activity? Do your periods or sexual relations cause you pain? Have you had children before? How did your previous pregnancies turn out? Have you ever had any abnormal Pap tests or sexually transmitted infections? How frequently do you get menstrual periods? Do you now or previously have any medical conditions? Do you come from a family with a history of health issues? Your doctor will be able to create an examination and probable treatment plan just for you with the aid of these and many other queries. A thorough history and a physical examination may also be done.

2)Transvaginal ultrasound - Ultrasound is a useful technique for assessing the uterus, fallopian tubes, and ovaries' structural characteristics. Distal fallopian tube blockage, ovarian abnormalities including ovarian cysts, and uterine abnormalities like fibroids and polyps can all be seen with ultrasound. Transvaginal ultrasound also gives your doctor the chance to gauge the proportion of eggs that are actually accessible. The antral follicle count is a parameter that may be related to reproductive potential.

3)Laboratory testing - Your doctor can ask for certain blood tests based on the findings of the assessment mentioned above. Measuring blood levels of specific hormones like estradiol and FSH, which are connected to ovarian function and total egg counts; TSH, which evaluates thyroid function; and prolactin, a hormone that, if increased, can impact menstruation function, are the most popular of these tests.

4)Hysterosalpingogram (HSG) - This test is crucial for assessing the health of the fallopian tubes, uterine filling issues such fibroids and polyps, and uterine cavity scarring (Asherman syndrome). The HSG can surgically treat a number of uterine and tubal disorders.

5)Semen analysis - The major test to assess the male partner is the semen analysis. Four parameters are examined: 1) Semen volume: at least 1.5 to 2 ml is required. 2) Sperm concentration - a normal concentration should be at least 20 million sperm per 1 ml of semen. A lesser number may indicate a structural or hormonal issue resulting in insufficient semen production. A lower concentration might reduce the likelihood of becoming pregnant naturally; sperm motility, or movement, should be at least 50% in order for it to be considered normal. Less than 50% motility may seriously impair sperm's capacity to fertilize eggs without treatment; and The head, midpiece, and tail of the sperm are the three areas that are examined for morphology, or form. Any abnormality in those areas might be a sign of sperm activity that isn't normal, which would make it more difficult for sperm to fertilize eggs. The capacity of sperm to fertilize the egg is best served by having between 5 and 15% of normal forms, according to stringent morphological requirements. A reproductive urologist should do a second assessment in the event that the semen analysis is abnormal. If necessary, your doctor will recommend that you see a reproductive urologist.

Chapter 2

Causes of infertility
If you've tried for a year to become pregnant and haven't been successful, you've been diagnosed with infertility. If you are a woman over 35, it signifies that you have tried becoming pregnant for six months and have been unsuccessful.

A woman may also be diagnosed with infertility if she is able to conceive but is unable to carry a pregnancy to term.

One who has never been able to conceive will be given the diagnosis of primary infertility. A woman who had at least one previous successful pregnancy will be given a secondary infertility diagnosis.

The issue of infertility affects men and women equally. Infertility can also affect men. In actuality, both men and women are just as prone to experience reproductive issues.

Approximately one-third of infertility cases can be attributed to female infertility, while another third of infertility cases can be attributed to issues with men, according to the Office on Women's HealthTrusted Source.

A combination of male and female infertility may be to blame for the remaining third of cases, or there may be no known cause.

Causes of infertility in male

Infertility in men typically results from problems with the following:

- Efficient sperm production:
- Sperm count, also known as the quantity of sperm,
- Shape of the sperm, and
- Movement of the sperm, which refers to both the sperm's own wriggling and the movement of the sperm through the male reproductive system's tubes.

Numerous risk factors, illnesses, and drugs can also have an impact on fertility.

Risk factors of infertility in males

Men's infertility is at risk for a variety of factors, including but not limited to:

- Cigarette smoking in senior age
- Excessive alcohol consumption obesity or overweight exposure
- Pollutants including pesticides, herbicides, and heavy metals
- Medical issues

Medical issues that can lead to infertility in males

- Testicles that haven't descended into the scrotum
- Having antibodies that target and kill your sperm
- A hormonal imbalance, such as low testosterone production
- Enlargement of the veins surrounding the testicles

Drugs and medications

Male fertility can also be impacted by a number of treatments and pharmaceuticals, including:

- Chemotherapy or radiation therapy for cancer
- Sulfasalazine (Azulfidine, Azulfidine EN-Tabs) for rheumatoid arthritis (RA) or ulcerative colitis (UC)
- Calcium channel blockers for high blood pressure
- cyclic antidepressants for depression
- Anabolic steroids for hormonal issues like delayed puberty
- Marijuana and cocaine for recreational use.

Conclusion

Infertility in men may result from any of these factors, or even from a combination of them.

Causes of infertility in women

Numerous variables that have an impact on or interfere with the following basic processes might lead to female infertility in women:

Fertilization takes place when the sperm and egg meet in the fallopian tube after passing through the cervix, and uterine implantation takes place when the fertilized egg attaches to the lining of the uterus where it may grow and develop into a baby.

Risk factors of infertility in females

The following are risk factors for female infertility:

- Cigarette smoking when one gets older
- Excessive alcohol usage
- Being substantially underweight, overweight, or obese having specific STIs that can harm the reproductive system

Medical issues that can lead to infertility in female

Infertility in women can be brought on by a number of medical problems that impact the female reproductive system.

Examples comprise:

- Ovulation abnormalities, which can be brought on by hormonal imbalances or polycystic ovarian syndrome (PCOS),
- inflammation of the pelvis (PID)
- Uterine fibroids and endometriosis
- Scarring from a prior operation caused by premature ovarian failure

Drugs and medications

Medications and substances that may have an impact on female infertility include:
- Radiation treatment or chemotherapy
- Antipsychotic medicines with long-term high-dosage nonsteroidal
- Anti-inflammatory drug (NSAIDS) usage, including aspirin (Bayer) and ibuprofen (Advil, Motrin).
- Recreational substances like cocaine and marijuana

The conclusion

Around one-fourth of couples' infertility difficulties are caused by ovulation abnormalities, according to the Mayo Clinic. Two indications that a woman may not be ovulating are an irregular menstruation or no period at all.

Chapter 3

Symptoms of infertility

It's typical for couples to face challenges with infertility. Many of these relationships are symptomless. Before they begin trying to get pregnant, they have no reason to believe they may suffer infertility.

Due of this, it is advised that couples who have been trying to conceive for more than a year without success consult a doctor. That time frame is shortened to six months for women over the age of 35. Age-related infertility problems get worse.

Infertility Symptoms and Signs

Infertility's signs and symptoms are frequently connected to other underlying illnesses. For instance, 10 to 15 percent of instances of untreated chlamydia will result in pelvic inflammatory disease (Trusted Source) (PID). PID causes the fallopian tubes to become blocked, preventing conception.

Both men and women can have infertility due to a variety of issues. Each one's warning signals and symptoms might differ substantially. It's crucial to speak with your doctor if you're worried.

These are some of the typical signs of infertility.

Common Symptoms of Female Infertility

1. Unusual cycles

The typical woman's cycle lasts 28 days. But as long as those cycles are regular, anything within a few days of that may be regarded as normal. A woman who has a 33-day cycle one month, a 31-day cycle the next, and a 35-day cycle the following month, for instance, is most likely experiencing "regular" periods.

However, irregular periods occur in a woman whose cycles are so unpredictable that she is unable to predict when she will have her period. This may be caused by polycystic ovarian syndrome or hormonal problems (PCOS). These two things both affect fertility.

2. Prolonged or painful periods
During their periods, most women feel cramps. However, painful periods that disrupt your everyday life might be an indication of endometriosis.

3. No commas
Women occasionally experience a bad month, which is common. Your menstruation may briefly stop due to stress or strenuous exercise. However, if it has been months since your last period, it is important to get your fertility examined.

4. Signs of fluctuating hormone levels
Women's hormone swings may be a sign of possible reproductive problems. If you encounter any of the following, speak with your doctor:
skin problems
Reduced sex is a factor in weight gain, thinning hair, and facial hair development. Sexual discomfort
Some women have believed that painful sex is normal since they have had it their entire lives. Yet it isn't. It could be connected to endometriosis, hormonal problems, or other underlying diseases that may possibly be causing infertility.

Common Symptoms of Male Infertility 1. Alterations in Sexual Desire
The health of a man's hormones is also related to his fertility. Changes in virility, which are frequently regulated by hormones, may be a sign of problems with conception.

2. Achy or painful testicles
There are several disorders that can cause discomfort or swelling in the testicles, and many of them can affect fertility.

3. Issues with keeping an erection

Hormone levels and a man's capacity for erection maintenance are frequently related. Reduced hormone levels might ensue, which might make it harder to get pregnant.

4. Problems ejaculating

Similar to the last example, it may be necessary to see a doctor if you are unable to ejaculate.

5. Tiny, solid testicles

In order for a guy to be fertile, the health of his testicles is essential. A doctor should investigate any potential problems that might be indicated by small or hard testicles.

Chapter 4

Treatment for Infertility

Couples can frequently still conceive even when a natural pregnancy does not occur by using assisted reproductive technologies. Treatment for infertility may require tremendous time, effort, and financial obligations.

Treatment of infertility in male

Men may receive the following treatments for general sexual issues or a shortage of good sperm:

- Adapting lifestyle elements.
- Changing one's lifestyle and engaging in certain behaviors, such as quitting some medications,
- Abstaining from harmful substances
- Increasing the frequency and timing of sexual activity
- Engaging in regular exercise, and optimizing other elements that might otherwise reduce fertility, can increase the likelihood of getting pregnant.
- Medications. A successful pregnancy may be more likely and sperm count may increase as a result of several drugs. These drugs may improve sperm quality and production as well as testicular function.
- Surgery. Surgery may be able to remove a sperm barrier and restore fertility in some cases. In some situations, surgically treating a varicocele could increase a woman's overall probability of getting pregnant.
- sperm extraction. When ejaculation is difficult or there are no sperm in the ejaculate, these methods can help. In situations when assisted reproductive procedures are intended but sperm counts are low or otherwise aberrant, they may also be employed.
- prostate biopsy. This is done for guys whose sperm counts are very low or nonexistent. If a guy is producing healthy sperm, a testicular biopsy with a needle might reveal this. If a testicle has a lot of healthy sperm, there is probably some sort of obstruction.

- Genetic analysis and Genetic testing can pinpoint particular sperm and infertility issues. The best time to do genetic testing is debatable among experts.

The creation of a pregnancy is the ultimate aim of therapy for male infertility. Ideally, the infertility's underlying cause may be treated, allowing for normal intercourse to lead to pregnancy.

Typical therapies for male infertility.

- The aberrant veins are blocked off during surgery to treat varicoceles. The fertility appears to significantly improve as a result, despite research to the contrary.
- Surgery or medication may be used to correct hormonal imbalances sometimes.

Sometimes, sperm transport plumbing obstructions can be surgically fixed.

In the past, male infertility was frequently permanent if the aforementioned treatments didn't succeed. Nowadays, significant new alternatives are provided by assisted reproductive technologies (ARTs).

These sophisticated and pricey therapies for male infertility offer sperm an artificial advantage over an egg. Even guys with very little or defective sperm can now become pregnant thanks to ARTs.

First, sperm are extracted from the testis with a needle or from ejaculated semen. After that, they go through many processes before being added to eggs.

- Implantation intrauterine (IUI.)

During ovulation, sperm are immediately delivered into the uterus. The ladies are typically administered medications initially to boost the quantity of eggs they produce.

In-vitro conception (IVF.)

Multiple eggs taken from the woman are combined with sperm in a "test tube" (actually just a plastic dish.). The uterus is then filled with fertilized eggs. IVF needs at least a few sperm that are viable.

- Injection of intracytoplasmic sperm (ICSI.)

A single sperm is put into an egg using a very small needle. After that, the fertilized egg is placed inside the uterus. When sperm counts are abnormally low or low, ICSI might be used.

According to Shaban, "most couples may expect a pregnancy between 40 and 50% of the time" while utilizing ARTs for several months.

Home remedies for infertility in males

Are there any actions you may do on your own to increase your fertility, though? Yes. Don't do anything that might reduce your ability to produce viable sperm, such as using marijuana, cocaine, cigarettes, or drinking more than two alcoholic beverages every day,

According to Shaban, using testosterone or any other over-the-counter androgen, such as DHEA (for weight training), might damage fertility.

Traditionally, infertility has been seen as a female issue. However, it turns out that males don't get away with it so simply. We are somehow implicated in infertility around half the time, and roughly one in every three cases of infertility is caused by the male alone.

One of the most difficult situations a guy may experience is receiving a diagnosis of male infertility. It may be disastrous for some people. After all, one of the few topics on which Darwin and the Bible concur is the requirement of reproduction. Guys who are unable to father a kid may feel as though they have failed in one of their most fundamental duties.

Unfortunately, some men must accept the fact that there is little they can do to treat their infertility. However, improvements in the management of male infertility are a tremendous aid for other men.

Testicles are where sperm are produced. The epididymis, which is a yard of "plumbing" that sits above each testicle, is where they are then kept. Semen, which is produced along the route by glands, feeds the sperm. When the miracle happens, a half-teaspoon of semen containing roughly 150 million sperm is ejaculated through the penis.

The success of the entire process depends on healthy amounts of testosterone and other hormones, as well as accurate nerve system signals.

Every month, women ovulate, or send an egg into the uterus. About 14 days after menstruation, this occurs. Pregnancy can be caused by sex at any point during the five days before to ovulation. Conception cannot occur during any other sexual activity, not even the day after ovulation.

According to Lawrence Ross, MD, president of the American Urological Association, "we normally urge couples to seek fertility assessments if they are unable to conceive after 12 months of unprotected intercourse." By that time, almost 85% of couples will have given birth. "After six months, if they are beyond 30, they should seek examination

Reasons for low sperm count in male

1)Varicocele, an abnormal cluster of protruding veins above the testicle, is the most prevalent factor in 38% of instances of treatable male infertility.

undescending sperm

infections that create a fever in the body, such as those that affect the testicles (orchitis), the prostate (prostatitis), or other organs

2)Cancer chemotherapy

drugs like anabolic steroids or seizure medications

anomalies in the genome

hormone issues

These issues can be fixed in some situations but not in others. The only way to figure things out is to have a doctor evaluate you.

Sometimes the issue is not sperm production. The challenge is getting the sperm to their intended destination. These male infertile men have healthy sperm in their testicles. However, the sperm in the semen are either defective, extremely few, or absent altogether. These factors contribute to this type of infertility:

3)Backward ejaculation In this circumstance, semen ejaculates into the bladder as opposed to the penis. The reason is typically past surgery.

absence of the vas deferens, the body's major sperm conduit. This disorder is caused by a genetic issue.

4)Obstruction. Anywhere in the plumbing between the testicles and the penis might have a blockage.

antibodies towards sperm. On their route to the egg, antibodies may inappropriately assault a man's own sperm.

5)Idiopathic infertility affects up to 25% of infertile males. That indicates that individuals have low or aberrant sperm levels for an unknown reason.

Treatment of infertility in females

Consult your doctor for assistance with the diagnosis and treatment of infertility if you haven't been able to conceive within an acceptable amount of time. A review of you and your companion is necessary. Your doctor will do a physical examination and collect a thorough medical history.

Examples of fertility testing

1)Testing for ovulation: The increase in luteinizing hormone (LH) that takes place just before ovulation is identified using an at-home, over-the-counter ovulation prediction kit. You may confirm that you're ovulating by having a blood test for the hormone progesterone, which is created after ovulation. Prolactin and other hormone levels may also be tested.

2)Hysterosalpingography. A procedure called hysterosalpingography (his-tur-o-sal-ping-GOG-ruh-fee) involves injecting X-ray contrast into your uterus and taking an X-ray to look for any issues there. The test reveals whether the fluid leaks from your fallopian tubes and leaves your uterus. If any issues are discovered, you'll probably want more testing.

3)Testing for ovarian reserve: The amount and quality of eggs accessible for ovulation are determined by this examination. These blood and imaging tests may be given to women who are at risk of having less eggs, such as those over 35.

4)Further hormone tests: Other hormone tests measure the levels of thyroid and pituitary hormones, which regulate reproductive processes as well as ovulatory hormones.

5)Imaging exams: A pelvic ultrasound test for fallopian tube or uterine cancer. Sonohysterograms, also known as saline infusion sonograms or hysteroscopies, can sometimes be utilized to reveal uterine characteristics that aren't visible on a standard ultrasound.

Occasionally, depending on your circumstances, your testing could involve:

6)Laparoscopy. In this minimally invasive procedure, your fallopian tubes, ovaries, and uterus are examined by inserting a thin viewing equipment via a tiny incision made beneath your navel. Endometriosis, scarring, blockages or abnormalities of the fallopian tubes, as well as issues with the ovaries and uterus, can all be found during a laparoscopy.

7)Genetic analysis Genetic testing assists in identifying any gene alterations that may be contributing infertility

Drugs to increase fertility

Fertility medications are medicines used to control or induce ovulation. The main form of therapy for women who are infertile because of ovulation problems is fertility medication.

In order to cause ovulation, fertility medications often act similarly to the natural chemicals follicle-stimulating hormone (FSH) and luteinizing hormone (LH). In order to attempt to induce a better egg or an additional egg or eggs, they are also utilized by women who ovulate.

Some fertility medications are:

1)Citrate of clomiphene: By stimulating the pituitary gland to generate more FSH and LH when taken orally, this medication promotes ovulation by encouraging the development of an ovarian follicle that contains an egg. In most cases, this is the first line of therapy for women under the age of 39 without PCOS.

2)Gonadotropins: These intravenous therapies encourage the ovary to release many eggs. Human menopausal gonadotropin, or hMG (Menopur), and FSH are examples of gonadotropin-containing drugs (Gonal-F, Follistim AQ, Bravelle).

3)Human chorionic gonadotropin (Ovidrel, Pregnyl): A different gonadotropin, is used to develop the eggs and cause their release at the time of ovulation. There are worries that using gonadotropins increases the risk of multiple pregnancies and preterm deliveries.

4)Metformin: This medication is utilized, often in PCOS-diagnosed female patients, when insulin resistance is a known or suspected contributing factor to infertility. Improved insulin resistance increases the chance of ovulation, which is improved by metformin (Fortamet).

5)Letrozole: Letrozole (Femara) functions similarly to clomiphene and is a member of the family of medications known as aromatase inhibitors. For PCOS, letrozole is often prescribed to women under the age of 39.

6)Bromocriptine.:A dopamine agonist called bromocriptine (Cycloset, Parlodel) may be used to treat ovulation issues brought on by the pituitary gland's excessive synthesis of prolactin (hyperprolactinemia).

Fertility medication dangers

Use of reproductive medications entails several dangers, including:

1)A multiple pregnancy :Less than 10% of multiple births are caused by oral drugs, and twin pregnancies are the majority of the time. Injectable drugs improve your odds by up to 30%. The substantial risk of triplets or more is also present with injectable fertility drugs.

Generally speaking, the risk of early labor, low birth weight, and developmental issues down the road increases with the number of fetuses you are carrying. The chance of multiples can occasionally be reduced by changing drugs if too many follicles emerge.

2)Syndrome of ovarian hyperstimulation (OHSS).:OHSS, which is uncommon, can result after the injection of reproductive medications to stimulate ovulation. Swollen and uncomfortable ovaries are one of the signs and symptoms, along with minor abdomen discomfort, bloating, nausea, vomiting, and diarrhea. These signs and symptoms often go away on their own.

A more severe form of OHSS that can also lead to fast weight gain, swollen, uncomfortable ovaries, fluid in the belly, and shortness of breath is also a possibility.

3) Ovarian Tumor Hazards throughout the long run: The majority of research on women who use reproductive medications points to little to no long-term harm. However, some research indicates that women who use fertility

medications for 12 or more months without conceiving successfully may be more likely to develop borderline ovarian cancers in later life.

Ovarian tumors are more common among women who have never been pregnant, therefore the cause may not be the therapy but rather the underlying issue. Reassessing drug use every few months and focusing on the therapies that have the highest success rates seem acceptable because success rates are often greater in the first few treatment cycles.

Operation to Regain Fertility

Several surgical treatments can boost female fertility by fixing issues or in other ways. However, due to the success of alternative therapies, surgical procedures for infertility are now uncommon. They consist of:

1)Either Hysteroscopic or Laparoscopic surgery: The uterine anatomy may need to be corrected surgically, endometrial polyps and some forms of fibroids that deform the uterine cavity may need to be removed, and pelvic or uterine adhesions may also need to be removed.

2)Tubal ligations: Your doctor could advise laparoscopic surgery to remove adhesions, widen a tube, or construct a new tubal opening if your fallopian tubes are obstructed or packed with fluid. This procedure is uncommon since in vitro fertilization often results in higher pregnancy rates (IVF). Your chances of getting pregnant with IVF after this operation may be increased by having your tubes removed or by having the tubes near to the uterus blocked.

Reproductive support

The most widely practiced reproductive aid techniques are as follows:

1)Implantation intrauterine (IUI):Millions of healthy sperm are injected into the uterus during IUI at or near ovulation.

technique for assisted reproduction. This entails taking mature eggs, fertilizing them with sperm in a dish in a lab, and then placing the fertilized embryos in the uterus. The most successful assisted reproductive method is IVF. Multiple blood tests and daily hormone injections are necessary throughout an IVF cycle, which takes many weeks.

Questions to ask your physician

 If we want to get pregnant, how frequently and when should we have sex?

Can we alter our lifestyles to increase our chances of getting pregnant?

Would you advise testing? What sort, if any?

Do any drugs exist that might increase a woman's chances of getting pregnant?

What negative effects may the drugs have?

Could you go through the specifics of our available therapy options?

What course of action would you suggest for us?

What percentage of couples you help become pregnant with success?

Do you have any printed materials, such as brochures, that we may borrow?

What websites would you suggest?

Feel free to ask any other questions you may have.

What to anticipate from your physician

Your doctor or another healthcare professional could ask you the following possible questions:

How long have you been attempting to conceive?

When was the last time you had sex?

Have you ever had a child? If so, how did the pregnancy turn out?

Have you undergone abdominal or pelvic surgery?

Have you ever received treatment for gynecological issues?

What age did you first have periods?

How many days, on average, elapse between the start of one menstrual cycle and the start of the following one?

Do you experience breast soreness, stomach bloating, or cramps as premenstrual symptoms?

Conclusion

Infertility treatment depends on the cause, your age, how long you've been infertile and personal preferences. Because infertility is a complex disorder, treatment involves significant financial, physical, psychological, and time commitments.Treatments can either attempt to restore fertility through medication or surgery or help you get pregnant with sophisticated technique Infertility treatment depends on the cause, your age, how long you've been infertile and personal preferences. Because infertility is a complex disorder, treatment involves significant financial, physical, psychological, and time commitments.

Treatments can either attempt to restore fertility through medication or surgery or help you get pregnant with sophisticated techniques.